YOUR KNOWLEDGE HAS VALUE

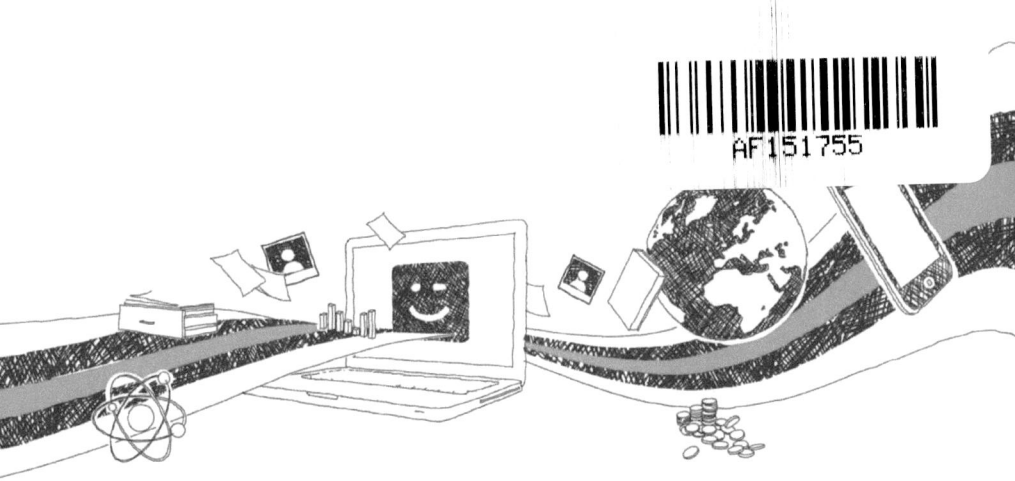

- We will publish your bachelor's and master's thesis, essays and papers

- Your own eBook and book - sold worldwide in all relevant shops

- Earn money with each sale

Upload your text at www.GRIN.com and publish for free

GRIN

Leonard Kabongo

Malaria and Anaemia: A Retrospective Case control study in a remote hospital in Zambia

GRIN Publishing

Bibliographic information published by the German National Library:

The German National Library lists this publication in the National Bibliography; detailed bibliographic data are available on the Internet at http://dnb.dnb.de .

Imprint:

Copyright © 2010 GRIN Verlag, Open Publishing GmbH
Print and binding: Books on Demand GmbH, Norderstedt Germany
ISBN: 978-3-640-90938-4

This book at GRIN:

http://www.grin.com/en/e-book/171547/malaria-and-anaemia-a-retrospective-case-control-study-in-a-remote-hospital

GRIN - Your knowledge has value

Since its foundation in 1998, GRIN has specialized in publishing academic texts by students, college teachers and other academics as e-book and printed book. The website www.grin.com is an ideal platform for presenting term papers, final papers, scientific essays, dissertations and specialist books.

Visit us on the internet:

http://www.grin.com/

http://www.facebook.com/grincom

http://www.twitter.com/grin_com

LEONARD KABONGO TSHIBASU

ID: UM12622HPU19937

FUNDEMENTALS OF EPIDEMIOLOGY

MALARIA AND ANAEMIA

A RETROSPECTIVE CASE CONTROL STUDY IN A REMOTE HOSPITAL IN

ZAMBIA

ATLANTIC INTERNATIONAL HOSPITAL

HONULULU HAWII

DECEMBER 2010

CONTENTS

1. INTRODUCTION

1.1. Situation analysis

Malaria is an endemic disease in Zambia and it's a major public health problem in Africa, especially in the Tropics and developing countries. Malaria continues to place an unacceptable burden on health and economic development in over 100 countries across the world, with malaria mortality exceeding one million annually, primarily in children under five(3).

Efforts have been put in place over the years to reduce the high incidence and mortality rate due to Malaria. From pharmaceutical options reviews to environmental actions, governments and their stakeholders through the Ministries of Health in various countries affected by the endemic, have worked to initiate policies for a massive and effective disease control.

According to WHO, about 109 countries in the world are considered endemic for malaria,45 countries within the African continent.3,3 billion people were estimated to be at risk of malaria in 2006.Of this total,2,1 billion were at low risk(<1 reported case per 1000 population),97% were living in regions other than Africa. The 1, 2 billion at high risk (≥1 case per 1000 population) were living mostly in the WHO African (49%) and South-East Asia regions (37%)(18).In the same report, there was an estimated death of 881,000(610,000-1,212,000) due to malaria in 2006, of which 91%were in Africa and 85% were of children under 5 years of age. (Table 1).

In Zambia, during a national malaria indicator survey, it was found that 22% of children below 5 years old of age had malaria. The highest malaria parasitemia were among children aged between 24-47 months. The distribution was higher in rural areas (28, 9%) than in urban areas (4, 9%). (9)

Table 1: Estimated of Malaria deaths by WHO region, 2006

Death(thousands)	Reported(all ages)	Reported(%<5 years)	Estimated(all ages)
Africa	156	88	801
Americas	0	29	3
Eastern Mediterranean	2	76	38
Europe	0	0	0
South-East Asia	2	35	36
Western Pacific	1	40	4
World	161	85	881

1.2. Objectives:

In this study, we would like to measure the magnitude of Malaria infection in line with the Fundamentals of Epidemiology. The objectives in this case control study is:

- To understand the epidemiological determinants of malaria associated with anaemia.

- To present and discuss epidemiologic elements in case control study

   (Magnitude of anaemia in malaria cases).

- To present a data analysis of the available data collected.

- Analyze the effectiveness of prevention and control measures.

The study is conducted at Sichili Mission Hospital, a remote hospital situated in Sesheke district at 287km from Sichili mission hospital is a first level referral hospital in the district. With 68 beds capacity, it is the only hospital in an area of 17,000 square kilometers with estimated population of 36,412(2009).
The Hospital is organized into 5 major in-patients department, out patients departments and paramedical services. The Male ward admits all male surgical and medical conditions. The female ward admits all female surgical, medical and gynecologic cases. The maternity ward admits all ante partum and postpartum patients and neonatology. The paediatric ward admits all children with various conditions. The Isolation ward admits all patients with Tuberculosis and mental illness. The theatre is functioning 24hourly for emergency cases and twice in week for elective operations.
Paramedical services available are physiotherapy, laboratory, and pharmacy.

1.3. Material and methods:

A retrospective case control study is conducted for 1 year (from January 2009 to December 2009) at Sichili Mission Hospital. Data is aggregated from in-patients medical files, OPD registries, Maternity registries, Laboratory reports and hospital annual reports.
Cases are defined as all patients who presented at the hospital with presumptive malaria symptoms and developed anaemia. Malaria was confirmed by thick and thin films of finger prick blood smears (11).
The controls are defined as all patients with same variables like cases, who presented at the hospital with symptoms suggestive of other illnesses but screened deliberately for malaria parasitaemia and were fund negative but had anaemia.
Patients whose blood smear was not collected were not included even though they were admitted.
Patients referred from the Rural Health centers to the hospital were considered, yet data from the center itself was not analyzed. The RHC (Rural Health center) use RDT (Rapid Diagnostic Test) for rapid and easy way for malaria diagnosis.

2. EPIDEMIOLOGIC DETERMINANTS

2.1. Definition:

Malaria is a protozoan disease caused by infection with parasites called 'Plasmodium" and transmitted to man by certain species of infected female anopheline mosquito (14). Malaria is a major cause of mortality and morbidity in the tropics and sub-tropical regions. (13)

2.2. Epidemiologic triad: Figure 1

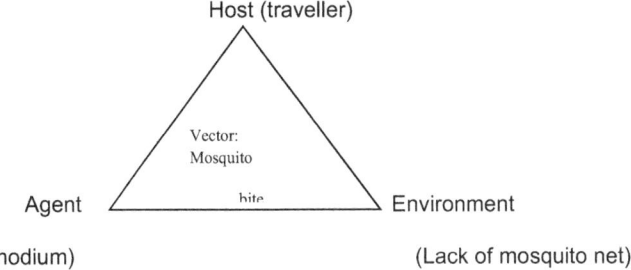

The above figure called the 'epidemiologic triad' shows the epidemiologic risk factors involved in the disease transmission. In Table 2, different factors are listed.

Table2: Risk and Protective factors

HOST	AGENT	ENVIRONMENT
Age,Sex,Race	Biological(bacteria)	Temperature
Religion	Chemical(poison)	Overcrowding
Occupation	Physical(trauma)	Neighbourhood
Marital status	Nutritional(Lack)	Housing
Education	Energy(thermal)	Radiation

2.2.1 Agent and Host

Four different species of Plasmodium parasite are responsible to cause malaria in humans: Plasmodium falciparum, Vivax, malariae and ovale.

In our region, plasmodium falciparum is mainly the cause of malaria morbidity and mortality. It's the most dangerous and, if untreated, causes cerebral malaria and death (10). The malaria parasite undergo 2 cycles of development: the human cycle (asexual cycle) and the mosquito cycle (sexual cycle).

The plasmodium multiplies in the anopheline gut and comes into its saliva glands each time the mosquito feed new blood (sporozoites). At the human bite, the sporozoites are transmitted into man and migrate to the liver where they multiply and destroy liver cells. Some merozoites of the ovale and vivax species will remain dormant in the hepatocytes (Hypnozoites) and will be responsible of Relapses.(16) After 9 to 15 days, the merozoites will be released in the blood stream and will colonize the erythrocytes. Here they enlarge and get a "ring form" (Trophozoites).This stage is accompanied by an active metabolism including the ingestion of the host cytoplasm and proteolysis of the haemoglobin in amino-acids. Mature scizonts (merozoites) are released following the rupture of the infected erythrocyte. The invasion of other erythrocytes initiates another cycle.

As an alternative to the asexual explicative cycle, the parasite can differentiate into sexual forms known as macro- or microgametocytes. The gametocytes are large parasites which fill up the erythrocyte, but only contain one nucleus. Ingestion of gametocytes by the mosquito vector induces gametogenesis (i.e., the production of gametes) and escape from the host erythrocyte.
Factors which participate in the induction of gametogenesis include: a drop in temperature, an increase in carbon dioxide, and mosquito metabolites.
Microgametes, formed by a process known as exflagellation, are flagellated forms which will fertilize the macrogamete leading to a zygote.
The zygote develops into a motile ookinete which penetrates the gut epithelial cells and develops into an oocyst. The oocyst undergoes multiple rounds of asexual replication resulting in the production of sporozoites. Rupture of the mature oocyst releases the sporozoites into the hemocoel (i.e., body cavity) of the mosquito. The sporozoites migrate to and invade the salivary glands, thus completing the life cycle.

In summary, malaria parasites undergo three distinct asexual replicative stages (exoerythrocytic schizogony, blood stage schizogony, and sporogony) resulting in the production of invasive forms (merozoites and sporozoites). A sexual reproduction occurs with the switch from vertebrate to invertebrate host and leads to the formation of the invasive ookinete. All invasive stages are characterized by the apical organelles typical of apicomplexan species. (7)

2.2.2. Environment

Malaria is widely spread in African regions, Asia and South America. The situation is worsened by multiple factors such as: poor or lack of health infrastructures to control the disease, long distances of populations to health facilities, erratic drug supply and political conflicts in regions with high prevalence. Outbreaks have been reported even in zones where the disease was under control.
Malaria is caused by an anopheline mosquito. There are almost 300 species of mosquitos, among them only 60 or so can transmit the infection. Male anopheles does not transmit the plasmodium as they feed only on plants juices.
Like all other mosquitos, the anopheline breed in water and have different preferred breeding grounds, feeding options and resting place.

2.3. Clinical manifestations:

Clinical manifestations of malaria include:
-Fever: This is the main symptom. Fever is generated by the subsequent release of merozoites (paroxysm) in the blood stream. Its characteristics vary according to the plasmodium species. Between the paroxysm time, patient feels well and the temperature is normal. Travellers who have never been exposed to the plasmodium before are tending to develop severe forms of malaria. For this reason, it is important to consider malaria in any person with fever who visited some malaria endemic zones recently (17).
-Other symptoms include joints pains or general body malaise, vomiting, body weakness, anaemia, delirium, confusion or loss of consciousness depending on the severity of the disease, the host immune system and genetics (19).

Severe forms of malaria which include cerebral malaria, hypoglycaemia, pulmonary edema, anaemia, renal failure, DIC (Disseminated Intravascular Coagulation), cyanosis.
Mostly these complications may constitute other research topics.
In this retrospective case control study, we are looking at the occurrence of anaemia in patients with malaria.

2.4 Treatment

According to WHO, the treatment of malaria requires more effort from governments to elaborate effective policies and implementation in the fight against the disease. Most of countries with high malaria incidence have tried not without success. The Zambian malaria initiative is one of the largest malaria control program which has proved tangible success in the region. In 2005, the National Malaria Control Program (NMCP) has set a goal of 75% reduction of malaria incidence and 20%reduction of under five mortality in 5 years through massive distribution of Insecticide Treated Nets (ITNs), Indoor residual spraying, Intermittent Preventive treatment of pregnant women using Sulphadoxine-Pyrimethamine,Use of Rapid Diagnostic Test and adopt Artemisinin-Based Combination as first line of malaria treatment. (12)

3. MALARIA INCIDENCE RATE

Malaria is associated with high mortality rate especially in children below 5 years of age. Half of the world's population is at risk of malaria and an estimated 243 million cases led to nearly 863 000 deaths in 2008. (20)
In this research paper, we analyzed the data of malaria associated with anaemia cases and controls for in patients and out patients from January 2009 to December 2009. (See Materials and methods).

The data is displayed in the next tables

Table 1: Malaria incidence rate in all age groups from January 2009 to December 2009.

Age groups	Malaria			Other illnesses			Total
	Female	Male	%	Female	Male	%	
0-1	14	14	14,8%	81	80	85,2%	189
1-4	60	46	21,1%	251	145	89,9%	502
5-14	200	140	60,7%	105	115	39,3%	560
15 and above	200	156	20%	711	715	80%	1782
Total	474	356	27,3%	1148	1055	72,7%	3033

Malaria cases among all consultations were higher in all age group with the highest among 5-14(60, 7% of all consultations in the age group).
Among the under 5 years, malaria represents almost 40 % of all consultations among the age group.
The incidence rate of malaria in 2009 at Sichili mission hospital is calculated as total malaria cases during the year divide by total population at risk during the same year.
Total population (all age):36,412

Incidence rate=$\frac{3033}{36,412} X 100 = 8,3\%$

Figure 1: Malaria incidence by age groups vs. other illnesses

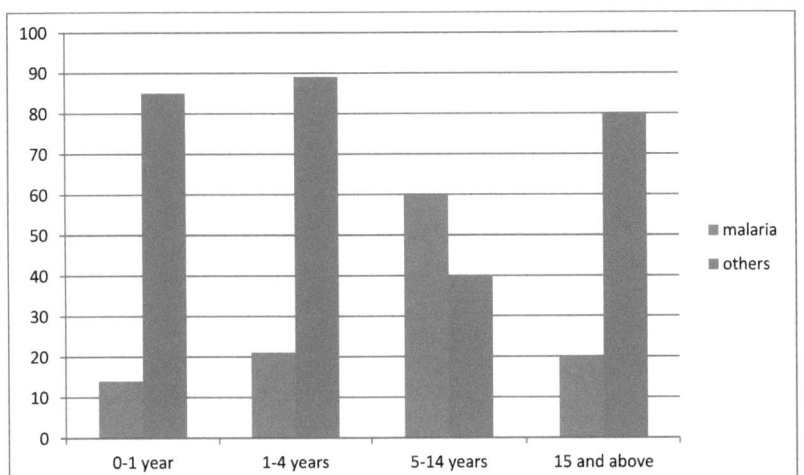

4. MALARIA AND ANAEMIA

In the context of malaria, anaemia is the common complication especially in children below 5 years of age and pregnant women. This hypothesis is been tested in a case control study. Malaria cases are defined as explained the section material and methods. Cases are patients diagnosed with marked anaemia (Hb<10g/dl). Controls are all patients who were diagnosed with anaemia related to other causes rather than malaria. Nevertheless, WHO expert group proposed that "anaemia or deficiency should be considered to exist" when haemoglobine (Hb) is below the following level (14). (See table 2).

In Zambia, Severe anaemia is considered as when the Hb≤6 g/dl and need blood transfusion as part of the management.

The following table shows the cut-off points for the diagnosis of anaemia.

Table 2:cut-off points for the diagnosis of anaemia

	g/dl Venous blood	MCHC (percent)
Adults male	13	34
Adults female non- pregnant	12	34
Adult female pregnant	11	34
Children 6 months to 5 years	11	34
Children 6 years to 14 years	12	34

4.1. Malaria and anaemia

The following table shows total anaemia cases for the period under review .n=163
Table 3: Anaemia cases

Age groups	male	female	total
0-4years	25	24	49
5-14 years	8	14	22
15 and above	42	50	92
total	75	88	163

The next histogram displays the same data

Figure 2: Total anaemia cases in different age groups.

Malaria with anaemia was high in both sex (92 cases) in adults (15 years and above).Nevertheless, 30 %(49) of all anaemia associated with malaria cases are children under 5 years of age. This value is significant and put children in this age category at risk.
The national malaria program strategy has got its means when targeting children under 5 as one of the risk population.
The next lines will be more practical with the fundamentals of epidemiology applied in this case-control review.

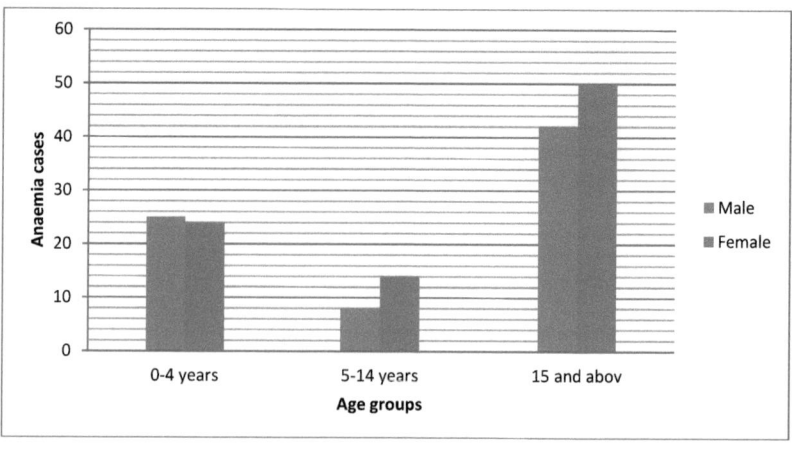

4.2. Odd ratio, relative risk and P-value

These epidemiological measurements are considered to test our hypothesis which is anaemia is the most seen complication of malaria in the tropics (especially in children below 5 years and pregnant women).For the sake of this study, pregnant constitute a special population and were not included.

This may be a research subject in future assignments.
The data has been displayed in different age categories (0-5years, 5-14 years and 15 and above) to major the statistical meaning of malaria associated with anaemia.

4.2.1. Malaria and anaemia in children below 5 years

The next 2x2 table represent the data for the cases (anaemia) and exposures (malaria) in children below 5 years.

Table 3: Case control study of malaria and anaemia for under 5 children at Sichili mission hospital in 2009.

Risk factors	Cases(Anaemia)	Controls(No anaemia)	total
Malaria	19(a)	115(b)	134
Other illnesses	30(c)	527(d)	557
Total	49	642	691

Exposure rates among the cases and the controls are given by the formulas below. Thus can be calculated as:
a. Cases=a/a+c=19/49=38, 7%

b.Controls=b/b+d=115/642=17,9%

4.2.2. Relative Risk (RR)

It clearly shown by exposure rates that the frequency rate of anaemia was higher among patients with malaria than among those without malaria.
The results above do not mean that among children exposed to malaria, 38, 7% will develop anaemia. For us to prove it, we need to calculate the Relative risk. This is given by a ratio between the incidence of disease among the exposed persons and the incidence of those not exposed.

Relative Risk= Incidence among exposed/incidence among non-exposed

$$= \frac{a}{(a+c)} / \frac{b}{(b+d)}$$

In general a relative risk can be only determined in a cohort study.
But in case control study, we can calculate an Odds ratio.

4.2.3. Odds ratio (cross product ratio)

The odds ratio is closed to the risk ratio and measures the strength of the association between the risk factors and outcomes.

Odds ratio=$\frac{\text{odds of exposure in those with the condition}}{\text{odds of exposure in those without the condition}}$

Recall that odds is calculated from a probability as

$$Odds = \frac{Probability}{1 - probability} \quad (15)$$

From the formula, Odds ratio will be given by

Odds ratio=ad/bc

In our study, Odds ratio=19x527/30x115=**2, 9**

This means children below the age of 5 with malaria have **2, 9** times risk of having anaemia than children with other illnesses.
To measure if this difference is statistical y significant, we have to calculate the P-value.

4.2.4. Calculation of P-value and implications

The P value is calculated to measure a "null hypothesis" that exposure is not related to disease. A higher P-value indicates that the data are highly consistent with the null hypothesis, and a low p-value indicates that the data are not very consistent with the null hypothesis (8). A set value of 0, 05 is the threshold for P-value. For instance if P-value is below 0, 05 it's regarded as statistically significant. The smaller the P-value, the greater the statistic significance.

How to calculate the p-value?
Consider the following risk data

	Exposed	Unexposed	Total
Cases	a	b	M1
Non cases	c	d	M2
People at risk	N1	N2	T

$$X = \frac{a - \frac{N1M1}{T}}{\sqrt{\frac{N1N2M1M2}{T^2(T-1)}}} = 3, 5$$

The p-value that corresponds to the x statistic must be obtained from the tables of standard normal distribution.
This x-value corresponds to a p-value of <0, 0001.
This value is statistically significant.
It should mean that children below the age of 5 with malaria are more likely to develop anaemia than those with other illnesses.
The result implies that the prevention of malaria would have a significant impact on the incidence of anaemia among children below 5 years. Thus, the malaria control program in various endemic countries is a considerable tool in the morbidity and mortality reduction.

Using the odds ratio or the P-value in different case control studies and cohort studies is a key indicator in the disease prognosis and treatment outcomes.
It is also essential to understand that odds ratio is not the same as relative risk, and relative risk is not the same as odds ratio. Both measure an association between a risk factor and an outcome, but relative risk is related to the difference in outcomes with and without a risk factor, and odds ratio is related to the difference in the presence of a risk factor in those with and without a condition.(15)

4.3 The control of confounding

The word "confounding" comes from the Latin "confundere", meaning to mix together. Confounding can have a very important influence, and may even change the apparent direction of an association. (1)
The control of confounding is necessary in a study to avoid biases in the result. For instance a protective variable may be revealed harmful after control of confounding. For a variable to be a confounder, it must, in its own right, be a determinant of the occurrence of disease (i.e. a risk factor) and associated with the exposure under investigation (5).
In our study pregnancy and malaria might present a confounding factor because malaria is a risk factor of anaemia as well as pregnancy. It was necessary to avoid the confounding factor by:
-Restriction: Cases and controls were selected strictly as malaria and non-malaria patients excluding pregnant women.
-Matching: Each patient with anaemia was selected in matching with the control in the same age group and sex to avoid confounding by age and sex.

Randomization, stratification and statistical modelling are other methods available to control confounding factor.

5. PREVENTION

Of all the malaria prevention modalities, bed nets suffer from the greatest problem in terms of a mismatch between distribution and effectiveness. The standard guideline is that every person living in a household not sprayed with indoor residual spraying should sleep under a bed net. However, utilization remains well below the 85% target. Some report sleeping under a bed net to be uncomfortably hot or claustrophobic, while others report irritation to the chemical treatments. There are also frequent reports of people not using nets at all, sometimes keeping them packaged as a sign of wealth or using them for other purposes (such as wedding veils and fishing nets), but there has been no systematic study to measure full utilization levels.
The other primary preventive intervention, indoor residual spraying (IRS), was carried out in 36 of Zambia's 72 districts in 2008, targeting primarily urban and peri-urban areas with relatively high population densities(4).
Treatment is another major component of the national malaria control program. The NMCC's strategic plan targets achieving "Prompt and Effective Case Management" (PECM), with a goal of ensuring that at least 80% of malaria patients receive effective treatment within 24 hours of the onset of symptoms. After noting decreasing

efficacy of Sulphadoxine/pyrimenthamine (SP) and chloroquine, Zambia became one of the first countries to introduce (specifically artemether plus lumefantrine, with the brand name Coartem®). ACTs, free in the public sector, became the first-line treatment for all malaria cases during the 2002-2003 malaria transmission season, but it wasn't until the 2005-2006 season that the drug reached all districts in the country. Until 2007 the country faced continuing challenges to retain national stocks. The national supply stabilized in 2007; since that time there have not been complete national stock-out periods, though logistical challenges in distribution to the provinces, districts and health facilities still remain (Sipilanyambe et al. 2008).

Basically, the Zambian malaria control strategy includes:
-The use of Insecticide treated Nets (ITNs)
-The Indoor Residual Spraying (IRS)
-The Intermittent Presumptive Treatment (IPT) to all pregnant women
-The use of Artemisinin-based combination therapy (ACT).
The Zambian malaria control strategy has been rated as one of the best malaria control program in high endemic malaria zones around the world.

The most important question would be how to prevent the maturation process of the parasite which happens under ecological and environmental conditions. The focus would be the control of environment and ecological determinant to successful control of malaria and its complications.
Being able to identify which ecological conditions are conducive to malaria transmission is an important step in being able to predict when malaria transmission is likely to occur and to effectively target malaria control. (6)

It has been shown that environmental and ecological factors are critical in the development to maturation of anopheles mosquitoes.
A minimal temperature of 18°C and a maximum of 40°C are favourable for the anopheline eggs to hatch. (2)

6. COCLUSION

Malaria being an endemic disease in Zambia and the leading cause of high morbidity and mortality rates. In the rural areas research has shown a high incidence rate than in the urban areas. The most affected people among the vulnerable are children below the age of 5 and pregnant women.
Prevention is a key to successful malaria control. Most of countries in endemic areas have implemented various program models to control the disease and its complications. One of the most commonly complication seen is anaemia.
Various epidemiologic fundamentals have been elucidated to understand the magnitude of malaria associated with anaemia in our setting. From epidemiologic triad, to measurements of relative risks, odds ratio-value and control of confounding, anaemia and malaria has shown a strong association especially in children below the age of 5 years in this case control study.
Thus the malaria control is vital in high endemic zones.
The Zambian malaria initiative has been seen as one of the successful malaria control program in the world.

The key in the global malaria control should include the following elements:
-The use of Insecticide Treated Nets (ITNs)
-The Indoor Residual spraying (IRS)
-The use of Intermittent Presumptive Treatment using Sulphadoxine-Pyrimethammine combination in pregnant women.
-The use of Artemisinin based combination therapy (ICT) as first line in the treatment of malaria and quinine in complication forms
The list is not exhaustive. Other methods especially environmental like temperature and sanitation may be considered where available and affordable.

REFERENCES

1. Bonita. R et all, Basic epidemiology, 2nd Ed, 2006

2. Cohen, J.M., et all, Topography-derived wetness indices are associated with household-level malaria risk in two communities in the western Kenyan highlands. Malaria Journal, 2008, page 7

3. GF report, Funding the Global fight against HIV/AIDS, Tuberculosis, Malaria, 2008-2009

4. Government of Zambia, Ministry of Health. National Malaria Control Action Plan: Actions for Scale-up for Impact on Malaria in Zambia. Lusaka.2008

5. Grimes DA, Schulz KF. Bias and causal associations in observational research. Lancet 2002; 359:248-52.

6. Gillian H.Stresman. Beyond temperature and precipitation: Ecological risk factors that modify malaria transmission, Elsevier 2010

7. http://www.tulane.edu/~wiser/malaria

8. Kenneth j.Rotman, Epidemiology, an Introduction, oxford University press, 2002

9. Ministry of Health, Zambian National malaria indicator survey, 2006

10. Microbiology byte journal, April 2009

11. Naseem Saba et all, outcome and complication of malaria in pregnancy, Gomal Journal of medical sciences July-dec 2008, vol 6 numb 2, pag 98-101

12. Nava Ashraf et all, Evaluating the effect of large scale health interventions in Developing country: the Zambian malaria initiative, National Bureau of Economic Research, June 2010, page 2-5

13. Osaro Erhabor et all, The prevalence of plasmodia parasitaemia among donors In the Niger delta of Nigeria, Tropical doctor, 2007, vol1, page 32-34

14. .Park K., Park's Textbook of Preventive and Social Medicine. 20th edition/s Banarsidas Bhanot.India.2009

15. Spiltalmic, Risk assessment 2, hospital physician, january2006, page 23-26, www.turner-white.com

16. White, NJ, Breman, JG. Malaria. In Harrisons Principles of Internal Medicine, 17th ed., McGraw Hill Co., New York, 2008:1280-1294

17. Wilson, et al. Fever in returned travellers: results from the GeoSentinel Surveillance Network. Clinical Infectious Disease 2007; 44:1560.

18. WHO, world Malaria report, 2008

19. WHO guidelines for the treatment of malaria. Geneva, World Health
Organization, 2006. http://www.who.int/malaria/docs/TreatmentGuidelines2006

20. WHO, Malaria report, 2009
www.who.int/malaria/world_malaria_report_2009/en/index.html